MENSTRUAL HEALTH & MANAGEMENT:

Empowering Women with Knowledge, Tools and Confidence for Every Cycle

By

Andrew Henri

i

TABLE OF CONTENTS:

Menstrual Health and Management

MENSTRUAL HEALTH AND MANAGEMENT

ACKNOWLEDGMENTS

Writing this book, **"Menstrual Health and Management,"** has been a deeply rewarding journey, and I am profoundly grateful to all those who have supported and inspired me along the way.

First and foremost, I extend my heartfelt gratitude to the pioneering authors whose groundbreaking work in the field of menstrual health has shaped my understanding and motivated me to embark on this endeavor. Dr. Jen Gunter, Dr. Christiane Northrup, and Dr. Aviva Romm, your insightful research, passionate advocacy, and dedication to women's health have been a constant source of inspiration. Your contributions have not only enriched my life but have also empowered countless individuals around the world to take charge of their menstrual health.

I would also like to express my deepest appreciation to my family for their unwavering support and encouragement throughout this journey. Your belief in me and your willingness to stand by my side through every challenge and triumph have been the cornerstone of my strength and resilience.

To my readers, I extend my heartfelt thanks for embarking on this journey with me. It is my sincere hope that this book serves as a valuable resource, empowering you to navigate your menstrual health with confidence, knowledge, and self-compassion.

Finally, I am immensely grateful to the countless healthcare professionals, activists, and advocates who tirelessly champion the cause of menstrual health and strive to create a world where menstruation is celebrated, not stigmatized. Your dedication and commitment to advancing menstrual equity and education are truly commendable, and I am honored to stand alongside you in this vital work.

With heartfelt gratitude,

Andrew Henri

DISCLAIMER

The information provided in this book, "Menstrual Health and Management: *Empowering Women with Knowledge, Tools, and Confidence for Every Cycle*", by Andrew Henri, is intended solely for educational and informational purposes. This book is not a substitute for professional medical advice, diagnosis, or treatment.

***Always seek the advice of your physician or other qualified healthcare provider with any questions you may have regarding a medical condition or treatment,** especially if you have any underlying health conditions.*

The authors and publishers of this book do not claim to diagnose, treat, cure, or prevent any medical conditions. The authors and publishers accept no responsibility for any adverse effects resulting from the use of the information contained herein.

The dietary, exercise and treatment recommendations in this book are general in nature and may not be suitable for everyone. It is important to tailor any recommendations to your individual needs and circumstances.
You are ultimately responsible for your own health and well-being.
This book is intended to be used in conjunction with the guidance of a qualified healthcare professional.
We encourage you to listen to your body and make adjustments to the recommendations in this book as needed.

INTRODUCTION:

EMBRACING YOUR MENSTRUAL HEALTH JOURNEY

Welcome to a transformative journey into the heart of understanding and managing your menstrual health. Whether you are just beginning to navigate the world of periods or seeking deeper knowledge to enhance your well-being, this book is designed to be your trusted companion. Menstrual health is not just about the days you bleed each month; it encompasses a spectrum of experiences, emotions, and physical changes that reflect the intricate balance of your body's natural rhythms.

For too long, menstruation has been shrouded in silence, surrounded by myths and misconceptions. It's time to break through these barriers and embrace a new narrative—one that celebrates and normalizes the menstrual cycle as an essential aspect of women's health. Understanding your menstrual cycle can empower you to make informed choices, enhance your quality of life, and foster a deeper connection with your body.

This book is more than just a guide; it's an invitation to explore, learn, and grow. We will embark on a comprehensive exploration of the menstrual cycle, delving into the biological, emotional, and practical aspects of menstruation. From recognizing the phases of your cycle to managing common symptoms and disorders, each chapter is crafted to provide you with valuable insights and actionable advice.

You will discover ways to maintain optimal menstrual health through nutrition, exercise, and self-care. You will find support in managing the emotional ups and downs that often accompany your cycle. You will learn about the latest menstrual products and innovations, as well as sustainable and eco-friendly options. Most importantly, you will gain the confidence to advocate for your health and well-being in every phase of life.

Together, we will challenge the stigma and taboos that have long surrounded menstruation, empowering you to talk openly and confidently about your experiences. By understanding and embracing your menstrual health, you can unlock a greater sense of control, comfort, and confidence.

So, let's begin this journey together. Open these pages with curiosity and a readiness to embrace the knowledge and tools that will help you thrive. Your menstrual health is a vital part of who you are—let's honor it, understand it, and manage it with the respect and care it deserves. Welcome to the journey of embracing your menstrual health.

Chapter 1:

Understanding Your Menstrual Cycle

1.1   What is a Menstrual Cycle?

The menstrual cycle is a natural, recurring process that prepares a woman's body for pregnancy. It involves a series of changes in the ovaries and the lining of the uterus, regulated by hormonal signals from the brain. Typically, the cycle is around 28 days long, but it can vary from 21 to 35 days in adults and from 21 to 45 days in young teens. Each cycle is unique and can be influenced by various factors, including stress, lifestyle, and overall health.

At its core, the menstrual cycle is a sign of reproductive health, but its importance extends beyond fertility. It is a window into your overall well-being, reflecting how different aspects of your life and health are in harmony or need attention. Understanding your menstrual cycle is crucial because it can help you recognize normal patterns and identify potential health issues early on.

🔊 *Call-to-Action:* Begin by observing and noting the regularity and characteristics of your menstrual cycle. This awareness is the first step towards taking control of your reproductive health.

1.2   Phases of the Menstrual Cycle

Cycle	Pre-ovulation		Ovulation	Post-ovulation
Ovarian cycle	Follicular phase			Luteal phase
Uterine cycle	Period	Proliferative phase		Secretory phase

The menstrual cycle is divided into four main phases: menstrual, follicular, ovulation, and luteal. Each phase is characterized by specific hormonal changes and physiological events.

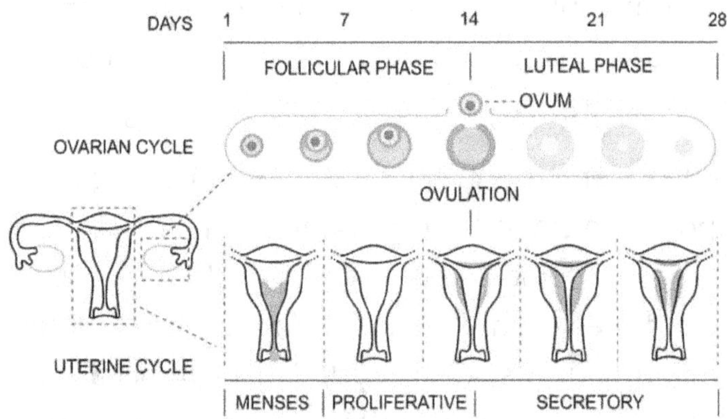

- ***Menstrual Phase (Days 1-5):*** This phase marks the beginning of the cycle. It starts on the first day of menstrual bleeding, which occurs as the uterine lining sheds. This phase typically lasts between 3 to 7 days. Hormone levels, particularly estrogen and progesterone, are at their lowest during this time, leading to the breakdown and expulsion of the uterine lining.

- ***Follicular Phase (Days 1-13):*** The follicular phase overlaps with the menstrual phase initially. During this phase, the pituitary gland releases follicle-stimulating hormone (FSH), which stimulates the ovaries to produce several follicles. Each follicle contains an egg, but usually, only one will mature fully. As the follicles develop, they secrete estrogen, which helps rebuild the uterine lining.

- ***Ovulation (Day 14):*** Ovulation occurs around the midpoint of the cycle, typically on day 14 of a 28-day cycle. A surge in luteinizing hormone (LH) triggers the release of the mature egg from the ovary. The egg then travels down the fallopian tube, where it may encounter sperm and become fertilized. This is the most fertile period of the cycle.

- ***Luteal Phase (Days 15-28):*** Following ovulation, the luteal phase begins. The empty follicle transforms into the corpus luteum, which secretes progesterone to maintain the uterine lining and prepare it for potential implantation of a fertilized egg. If fertilization does not occur, the corpus luteum breaks down, leading to a drop in progesterone and estrogen levels, and the cycle starts anew with the menstrual phase.

Understanding these phases can help you recognize the natural rhythms of your body and manage symptoms more effectively.

- 🔊 *Call-to-Action*: Reflect on your experiences during each phase of your cycle. Are there specific symptoms or changes in mood and energy that you notice? Keeping a journal can help you track these patterns.

1.3   Common Menstrual Cycle Variations

Not all menstrual cycles follow the textbook 28-day pattern. Variations are common and can be influenced by a range of factors. Here are some typical variations:

- **Irregular Cycles:** Cycles that vary in length by more than a few days each month can be considered irregular. Causes may include stress, significant weight changes, exercise, or underlying medical conditions such as polycystic ovary syndrome (PCOS).
- **Anovulatory Cycles:** Sometimes, a cycle may occur without ovulation. These anovulatory cycles can result in missed or irregular periods and may be influenced by factors like stress, hormonal imbalances, or significant weight fluctuations.
- **Short or Long Cycles:** Cycles shorter than 21 days or longer than 35 days may be normal for some women, but they can also indicate underlying health issues. For example, thyroid disorders or hyperprolactinemia (excessive production of prolactin) can cause longer cycles.
- **Heavy or Prolonged Bleeding:** Menorrhagia, or excessively heavy or prolonged menstrual bleeding, can be caused by conditions such as fibroids, endometriosis, or hormonal imbalances. It's essential to seek medical advice if you experience significantly heavy or prolonged periods.
- **Painful Periods:** Dysmenorrhea, or painful periods, can vary from mild discomfort to severe pain that interferes with daily activities. Causes can include primary dysmenorrhea (common menstrual cramps) or secondary

dysmenorrhea (due to underlying conditions like endometriosis or fibroids).

🔊 *Call to Action*: If you notice significant changes or irregularities in your menstrual cycle, don't hesitate to consult a healthcare provider. Early detection of potential issues can lead to more effective management and better overall health outcomes.

1.4   Tracking Your Cycle: Apps and Techniques

Tracking your menstrual cycle is an invaluable tool for understanding your body and managing your health. There are several methods and tools available to help you monitor your cycle accurately:

- **Menstrual Cycle Apps:** Several apps are designed to help women track their menstrual cycles, symptoms, and ovulation. Popular options include Clue, Flo, and Period Tracker. These apps allow you to log daily symptoms, moods, and physical changes, providing insights into patterns and predicting future cycles.
- **Basal Body Temperature (BBT):** Tracking your basal body temperature—your temperature when you first wake up—can help pinpoint ovulation. A slight increase in BBT typically indicates ovulation has occurred. Using a BBT thermometer, you can track these changes over time to identify patterns.
- **Cervical Mucus Monitoring:** The consistency and amount of cervical mucus change throughout the menstrual cycle. Monitoring these changes can help identify fertile days.

For example, during ovulation, cervical mucus is typically clear and stretchy, resembling egg whites.

- ***Calendar Method:*** This traditional method involves marking the first day of your period on a calendar and tracking the cycle length over several months. This method can be useful for identifying patterns and estimating future periods.
- ***Symptom Charting:*** Keeping a daily log of symptoms, such as cramps, mood changes, and energy levels, can help you understand how your cycle affects you physically and emotionally. This information can be invaluable when discussing menstrual health with your healthcare provider.
  - 🔊 *Call-to-Action*: Choose a tracking method that suits your lifestyle and start tracking your cycle today. Consistent tracking can provide valuable insights and help you take proactive steps towards better menstrual health.

Chapter 2:

Menstrual Health Essentials

Understanding the intricacies of the female reproductive system and the hormonal interplay that governs the menstrual cycle is crucial for managing menstrual health effectively. This chapter delves into the essential aspects of menstrual health, providing a comprehensive guide to the anatomy, hormonal dynamics, common disorders, and critical warning signs that require medical attention.

2.1   Anatomy of the Female Reproductive System

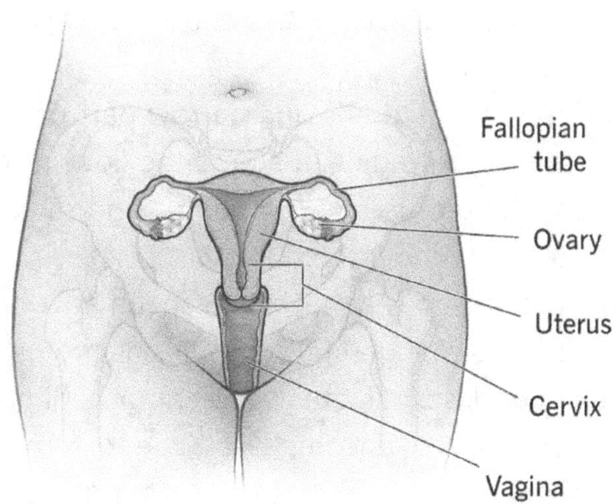

The female reproductive system is a complex network of organs that work together to regulate menstruation, facilitate reproduction, and maintain hormonal balance. Here's an overview of its key components:

- **Ovaries:** The ovaries are two small, almond-shaped organs located on either side of the uterus. They produce eggs (ova) and secrete hormones such as estrogen and progesterone. Each ovary contains thousands of follicles, each housing an immature egg.
- **Fallopian Tubes:** These narrow tubes connect the ovaries to the uterus. During ovulation, an egg is released from an ovary and travels down the fallopian tube, where fertilization by a sperm cell may occur.
- **Uterus:** The uterus is a pear-shaped muscular organ located in the pelvis. Its lining, the endometrium, thickens each month in preparation for a potential pregnancy. If fertilization does not occur, the endometrial lining sheds during menstruation.
- **Cervix:** The cervix is the lower, narrow part of the uterus that opens into the vagina. It allows the flow of menstrual blood from the uterus into the vagina and directs sperm into the uterus during intercourse.
- **Vagina:** The vagina is a muscular canal that connects the cervix to the external genitals. It serves as the passage for menstrual blood, sexual intercourse, and childbirth.
- **Vulva:** The vulva encompasses the external genital organs, including the labia majora and minora, clitoris, and vaginal opening. It plays a crucial role in sexual arousal and protection of internal reproductive organs.

📢 *Call-to-Action*: Familiarize yourself with your reproductive anatomy. Understanding how each part functions can empower you to recognize normal and abnormal changes in your menstrual health.

2.2   Hormones and Their Roles

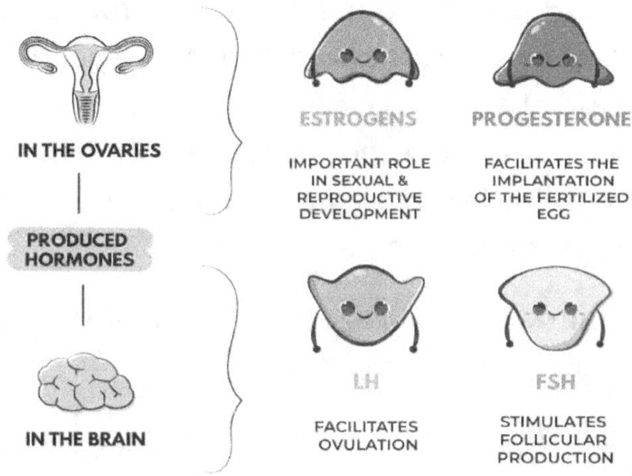

Hormones are chemical messengers that regulate various functions in the body, including the menstrual cycle. Key hormones involved in the menstrual cycle include:

- **Estrogen:** Produced primarily by the ovaries, estrogen is responsible for the growth and maintenance of the female reproductive system and secondary sexual characteristics. It helps regulate the menstrual cycle by thickening the endometrial lining during the follicular phase.

- **Progesterone:** After ovulation, the corpus luteum in the ovary produces progesterone. This hormone stabilizes the endometrial lining, preparing it for potential implantation of a fertilized egg. If pregnancy does not occur, progesterone levels drop, triggering menstruation.

- **Follicle-Stimulating Hormone (FSH):** FSH is produced by the pituitary gland and stimulates the growth of ovarian follicles during the follicular phase. It plays a critical role in the maturation of eggs.
- **Luteinizing Hormone (LH):** Also produced by the pituitary gland, LH surges mid-cycle to trigger ovulation—the release of a mature egg from the ovary.
- **Gonadotropin-Releasing Hormone (GnRH):** GnRH is secreted by the hypothalamus and regulates the release of FSH and LH from the pituitary gland.

Dr. Mary Jane Minkin, a clinical professor of obstetrics and gynecology at Yale University, explains,

"Understanding the hormonal changes that occur throughout your cycle can help you anticipate and manage symptoms more effectively. Hormones play a pivotal role in your overall health and well-being."

📢 *Call-to-Action*: Track your symptoms in relation to your cycle phases. Noting how your body responds to hormonal changes can help you better manage menstrual-related symptoms and communicate more effectively with your healthcare provider.

2.3   Common   Menstrual   Disorders: PCOS, Endometriosis, and More

Several menstrual disorders can impact your health and quality of life. Here are some of the most common conditions:

- ***Polycystic Ovary Syndrome (PCOS):*** PCOS is a hormonal disorder characterized by irregular menstrual periods, excess androgen levels, and polycystic ovaries. Symptoms include irregular cycles, acne, hirsutism (excess hair growth), and weight gain.

Dr. Fiona McCullough, a registered dietitian and author of *8 Steps to Reverse Your PCOS*, notes:

> *"PCOS is a complex condition that requires a comprehensive approach, including lifestyle changes, to manage effectively."*

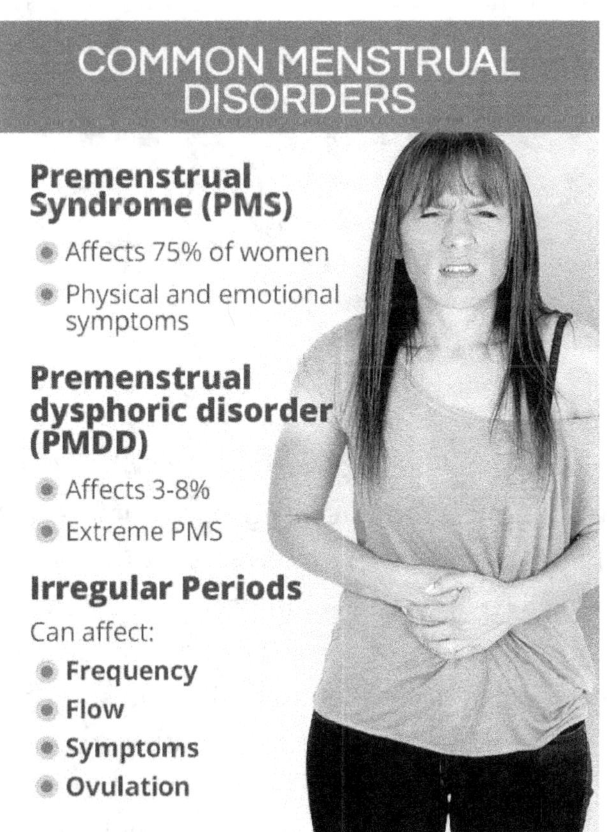

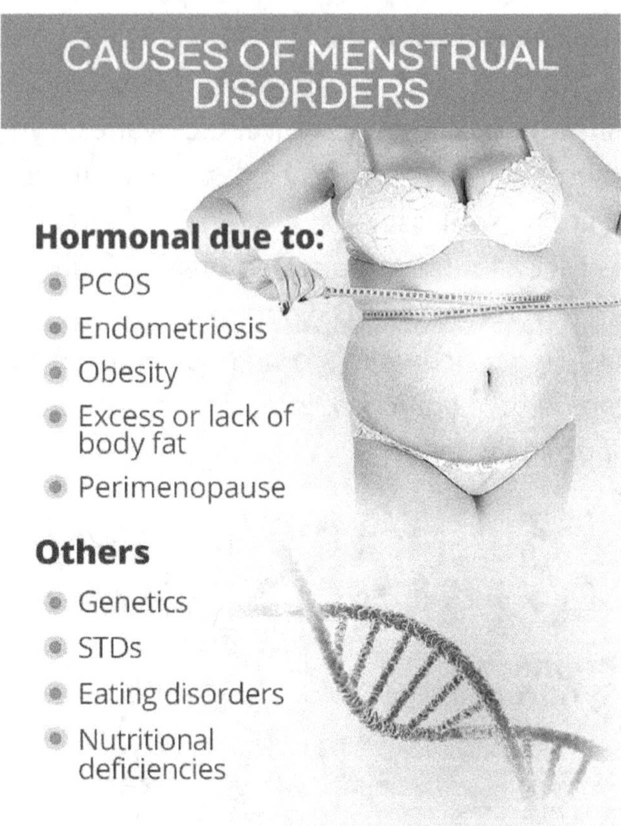

- ***Endometriosis:*** Endometriosis occurs when tissue similar to the lining of the uterus grows outside the uterus, causing pain and often infertility. Common symptoms include severe menstrual cramps, chronic pelvic pain, and heavy periods. Treatment options range from pain management to hormonal therapies and surgery.

- ***Fibroids:*** Uterine fibroids are non-cancerous growths in the uterus that can cause heavy menstrual bleeding, prolonged periods, and pelvic pain. While many fibroids are asymptomatic, those causing significant symptoms may require medical or surgical treatment.

- ***Premenstrual Syndrome (PMS) and Premenstrual Dysphoric Disorder (PMDD):*** PMS includes a range of physical and emotional symptoms occurring before menstruation. PMDD is a severe form of PMS with symptoms that can significantly disrupt daily life. Treatment options include lifestyle changes, medications, and therapy.
- ***Amenorrhea:*** Amenorrhea is the absence of menstruation. Primary amenorrhea refers to a delay in the onset of menstruation, while secondary amenorrhea is the cessation of periods after they have begun. Causes can include hormonal imbalances, stress, excessive exercise, and certain medical conditions.
    - 📣 *Call-to-Action*: If you experience symptoms of any menstrual disorder, seek medical advice. Early diagnosis and treatment can improve your quality of life and prevent complications.

2.4 When to See a doctor: Recognizing Warning Signs

Recognizing when to seek medical attention is crucial for maintaining menstrual health. Here are some warning signs that warrant a visit to a healthcare provider:

- ***Irregular Periods***: Significantly irregular cycles or changes in cycle length can indicate underlying health issues.

Consistently irregular periods should be evaluated by a healthcare professional.

- **Heavy or Prolonged Bleeding:** Menstrual bleeding that soaks through one or more sanitary products every hour for several consecutive hours or periods lasting longer than seven days can signal a problem.
- **Severe Pain:** While some discomfort is normal, severe menstrual cramps or pelvic pain that disrupts daily activities is not. This pain could indicate conditions like endometriosis or fibroids.
- **Absence of Periods:** Missing periods (amenorrhea) for three or more consecutive cycles, or not starting menstruation by age 16, should be evaluated.
- **Unusual Symptoms:** Symptoms such as excessive hair growth, unexplained weight gain, severe mood changes, or symptoms of menopause before age 40 (premature ovarian insufficiency) should prompt a medical consultation.

Dr. Carolyn Alexander, an obstetrician-gynecologist at Southern California Reproductive Center, emphasizes:

"It's important for women to listen to their bodies and seek medical advice when something feels off. Early intervention can make a significant difference in managing menstrual health issues."

- 🔊 Call to Action: Be proactive about your menstrual health. Regular check-ups and open communication with your healthcare provider can help you address concerns promptly and maintain optimal health.

Key Facts to Remember

✓ *Anatomy and Hormones:* Understanding the female reproductive system and hormonal roles is fundamental to managing menstrual health.

✓ *Common Disorders:* PCOS, endometriosis, fibroids, PMS, and amenorrhea are common menstrual disorders that can significantly impact quality of life.

✓ *Warning Signs:* Recognizing irregularities, heavy bleeding, severe pain, missed periods, and unusual symptoms is crucial for timely medical intervention.

By arming yourself with knowledge about your menstrual health, you can take charge of your well-being and make informed decisions that enhance your quality of life. This awareness empowers you to seek the right care, manage symptoms effectively, and maintain a healthy, balanced life.

Chapter 3:

Managing Menstrual Symptoms

Menstrual symptoms can vary widely in intensity and type, impacting women's daily lives in numerous ways. Effective management of these symptoms is essential for maintaining quality of life and overall well-being. This chapter explores various strategies for dealing with common menstrual symptoms, from cramps and heavy periods to PMS and PMDD, with an emphasis on both conventional and holistic approaches.

3.1 Dealing with Cramps: Home Remedies and Medications

Menstrual cramps, or dysmenorrhea, are a common complaint among women. They are caused by the contraction of the uterine muscles as they shed the lining during menstruation. For many, these cramps can range from mild discomfort to severe pain that disrupts daily activities. Here are effective ways to manage menstrual cramps:

Home Remedies for
Menstrual Cramp Relief

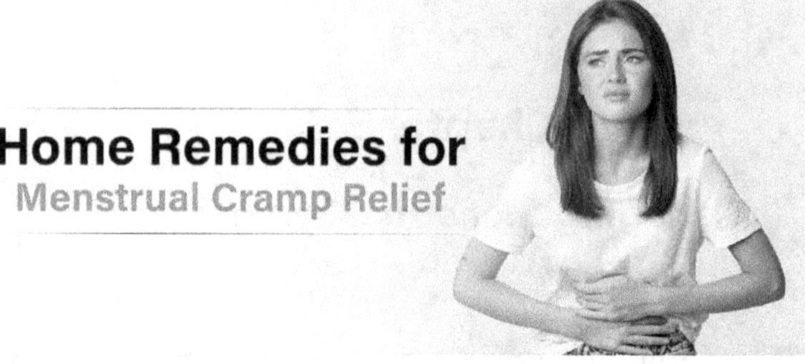

Home Remedies

- ***Heat Therapy:*** Applying heat to the lower abdomen can help relax the muscles and alleviate pain. Use a heating pad, hot water bottle, or take a warm bath. Dr. Jennifer Wider, a women's health expert, states, *"Heat therapy is a simple yet effective way to ease menstrual cramps. It increases blood flow and helps soothe the muscles."*
- ***Hydration:*** Staying hydrated can reduce bloating and ease cramping. Drinking warm liquids like herbal teas can be particularly soothing.
- ***Exercise:*** Light physical activity, such as walking or yoga, can increase blood flow and reduce cramp severity. Exercise releases endorphins, which act as natural painkillers.
- ***Dietary Adjustments:*** Eating a balanced diet rich in fruits, vegetables, and whole grains can help. Avoiding caffeine and salty foods can reduce bloating and water retention.

Medications:

- ***Over-the-Counter Pain Relievers:*** Nonsteroidal anti-inflammatory drugs (NSAIDs) like ibuprofen (Advil, Motrin) and naproxen (Aleve) are commonly used to relieve menstrual pain. These medications reduce the production of prostaglandins, chemicals that cause cramping.

- ***Prescription Medications:*** For severe cramps, a healthcare provider might prescribe stronger NSAIDs or hormonal treatments like birth control pills, which can regulate or even eliminate periods.

  - 📢 *Call to Action*: Keep a menstrual diary to track the severity of your cramps and the effectiveness of different treatments. This information can be helpful when discussing symptoms with your healthcare provider.

3.2 Managing Heavy Periods

Heavy menstrual bleeding, or menorrhagia, can significantly impact daily life and lead to anemia if not managed properly. Understanding and addressing the causes of heavy periods is crucial for effective treatment. Here are some strategies:

1. Medical Treatments:

- ***Hormonal Contraceptives***: Birth control pills, hormonal IUDs (such as Mirena), and contraceptive patches can help regulate periods and reduce bleeding. These methods work by thinning the uterine lining.

- ***Tranexamic Acid:*** This prescription medication helps reduce menstrual bleeding by aiding blood clotting. It's taken only during menstruation.

- ***Nonsteroidal Anti-Inflammatory Drugs (NSAIDs):*** NSAIDs not only reduce menstrual cramps but also decrease blood loss by reducing prostaglandin levels.
- ***Iron Supplements:*** If heavy bleeding leads to anemia, iron supplements can help restore proper blood levels. A healthcare provider can determine the appropriate dosage.

2. Surgical Treatments:

1. ***Endometrial Ablation***: This procedure destroys the lining of the uterus to reduce or stop menstrual bleeding. It's an option for women who do not plan to have more children.
2. ***Uterine Fibroid Embolization***: For heavy bleeding caused by fibroids, this procedure blocks blood flow to fibroids, causing them to shrink.
3. ***Hysterectomy***: In severe cases, removing the uterus may be considered, especially if other treatments have failed. This is a major surgery and eliminates the ability to become pregnant.
   - 🔊 *Call to Action:* If you experience heavy bleeding that interferes with your daily life or leads to symptoms of anemia (such as fatigue or shortness of breath), consult a healthcare provider. Keeping a record of your bleeding patterns can aid in diagnosis and treatment.

3.3   Coping with PMS and PMDD

Premenstrual Syndrome (PMS) and Premenstrual Dysphoric Disorder (PMDD) encompass a range of physical and emotional symptoms that occur in the luteal phase of the menstrual cycle. PMDD is a more severe form of PMS and can significantly impair daily functioning. Here's how to cope with these conditions:

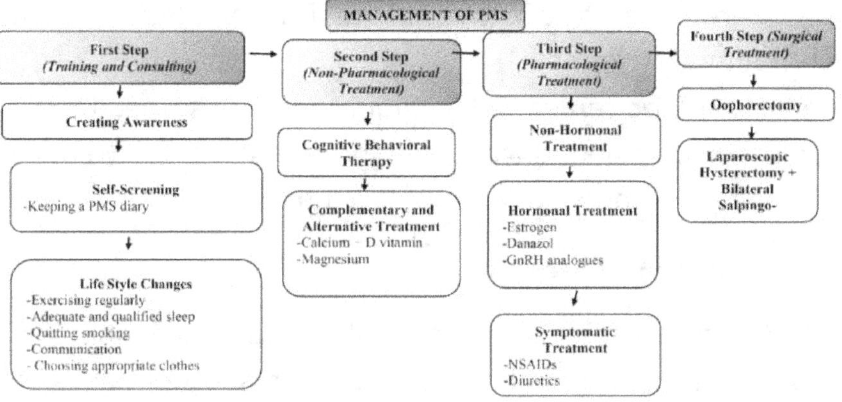

1. Lifestyle Adjustments:

- ***Diet and Nutrition***: Eating small, frequent meals rich in complex carbohydrates can stabilize blood sugar levels and reduce PMS symptoms. Limiting caffeine, sugar, and alcohol intake can also help.
- ***Regular Exercise:*** Physical activity, such as aerobic exercise, can boost mood and energy levels, reducing the severity of PMS and PMDD symptoms.
- ***Sleep Hygiene:*** Ensuring adequate, quality sleep is vital. Aim for 7-9 hours of sleep per night and maintain a consistent sleep schedule.

2. Psychological Strategies:

- ***Cognitive Behavioral Therapy (CBT):*** CBT can help manage the emotional symptoms of PMS and PMDD by addressing negative thought patterns and promoting healthier coping mechanisms. Dr. Marla Shapiro, a women's health expert, notes, "CBT is a valuable tool for managing the psychological impact of PMDD. It helps women develop effective strategies for dealing with emotional symptoms."

- **Stress Management:** Techniques such as meditation, mindfulness, and deep-breathing exercises can reduce stress and improve overall well-being.

3. Medical Treatments:

- **Antidepressants:** Selective serotonin reuptake inhibitors (SSRIs) are commonly prescribed for severe PMS and PMDD. They can help alleviate mood swings, depression, and anxiety.
- **Hormonal Treatments:** Birth control pills, hormonal IUDs, and GnRH agonists can help regulate hormonal fluctuations and reduce symptoms.
- **Supplements:** Certain supplements, such as calcium, magnesium, and vitamin B6, have been shown to alleviate PMS symptoms. Always consult with a healthcare provider before starting any new supplement regimen.
  - 📢 *Call to Action:* Track your symptoms using a menstrual diary to identify patterns and triggers. This can help you and your healthcare provider develop an effective management plan.

3.4   Natural and Holistic Approaches

Many women seek natural and holistic approaches to manage menstrual symptoms, either as a complement to conventional treatments or as a primary method. Here are some popular options:

1. Herbal Remedies:

- ***Chasteberry (Vitex):*** This herb is known for its ability to balance hormones and reduce symptoms of PMS. Studies have shown that chasteberry can be effective in alleviating breast tenderness, mood swings, and irritability.
- ***Ginger:*** Ginger has anti-inflammatory properties and can help reduce menstrual pain. Consuming ginger tea or supplements can provide relief.
- ***Evening Primrose Oil:*** Rich in gamma-linolenic acid (GLA), evening primrose oil is often used to reduce PMS symptoms, including breast pain and mood swings.

2. Acupuncture:

Acupuncture involves inserting thin needles into specific points on the body to relieve pain and promote healing. Some studies suggest that acupuncture can be effective in reducing menstrual pain and other PMS symptoms.

3. Mind-Body Techniques:

- ***Yoga:*** Practicing yoga can help reduce stress, improve flexibility, and alleviate menstrual cramps. Specific poses, such as the child's pose and the bridge pose, can be particularly beneficial.

- ***Meditation and Mindfulness:*** These practices can help manage stress and improve emotional well-being. Mindfulness meditation, in particular, has been shown to reduce symptoms of PMS and PMDD.

4. Dietary Supplements:

- ***Omega-3 Fatty Acids:*** Found in fish oil, flaxseeds, and chia seeds, omega-3 fatty acids have anti-inflammatory properties that can help reduce menstrual pain and improve mood.
- ***Magnesium:*** Magnesium supplements can help alleviate menstrual cramps and reduce symptoms of PMS. Foods rich in magnesium, such as leafy greens, nuts, and seeds, are also beneficial.
  - 🔊 ***Call to Action***: Explore natural and holistic approaches that resonate with you. Always consult with a healthcare provider before starting any new treatment to ensure it's safe and appropriate for your situation.

Key Facts to Remember

- ✓ *Managing Cramps*: Heat therapy, hydration, exercise, and NSAIDs are effective ways to alleviate menstrual cramps.
- ✓ *Heavy Periods*: Hormonal treatments, tranexamic acid, and surgical options can help manage heavy menstrual bleeding.
- ✓ *PMS and PMDD:* Lifestyle adjustments, CBT, stress management, and medical treatments like SSRIs can alleviate symptoms.

✓ *Natural Approaches*: Herbal remedies, acupuncture, yoga, and dietary supplements offer holistic options for managing menstrual symptoms.

By understanding and utilizing various strategies to manage menstrual symptoms, you can take proactive steps towards improving your menstrual health and overall quality of life. Each woman's experience is unique, so it's important to find the methods that work best for you and seek professional guidance when needed.

Chapter 4:

Menstrual Hygiene and Products

Maintaining good menstrual hygiene is essential for preventing infections, ensuring comfort, and promoting overall well-being. This chapter explores the variety of menstrual products available, best practices for menstrual hygiene, eco-friendly options, and innovations in menstrual care. Understanding these aspects can empower you to make informed choices that suit your lifestyle and health needs.

4.1   Choosing the Right Menstrual Products: *Pads, Tampons, Cups, and More*

Selecting the right menstrual product is a personal choice that depends on individual preferences, lifestyle, and menstrual flow. Here's an overview of the most common menstrual products:

1. Pads:

- *Definition:* Pads, also known as sanitary napkins, are absorbent materials worn inside the underwear to absorb menstrual blood. They come in various sizes and thicknesses, with or without wings (flaps that fold over the sides of underwear to keep the pad in place).

Pros:

- Easy to use and widely available.
- Suitable for all flow levels.
- No risk of Toxic Shock Syndrome (TSS), a rare but serious condition caused by bacterial toxins.

Cons:

- Can be bulky and visible under clothing.
- May cause discomfort or skin irritation if not changed regularly.

MENSTRUAL CLOTH	REUSABLE PAD	DISPOSABLE PAD	MENSTRUAL CUP	TAMPON
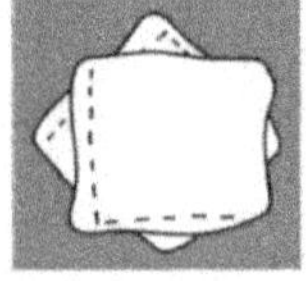	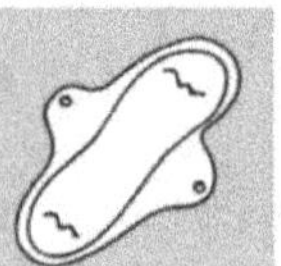	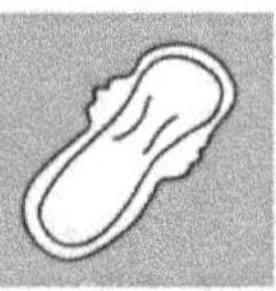	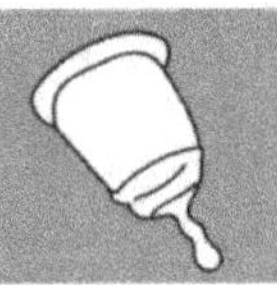	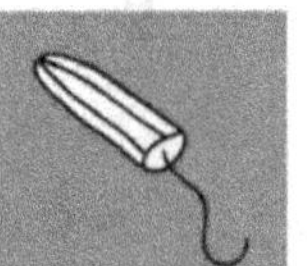
Reusable, affordable, already used in many contexts. Relies on privacy, clean water and soap, and time to wash and dry.	Reusable, can be home-made or produced locally, where good quality, comfortable. Relies on privacy, water soap and time to wash and dry.	Convenient, widely available, preferred by many women and girls, comfortable. Relies on disposal systems and access to markets.	Reusable, available in some countries. Relies on privacy, water and soap to clean, and hindered by cultural taboos on inserting and virginity.	Convenient, available in some countries. Relies on disposal systems and hindered by cultural taboos surrounding insertion and virginity.

2. Tampons:

- *Definition:* Tampons are cylindrical devices made of absorbent material that are inserted into the vagina to absorb menstrual blood. They come with or without applicators for insertion.

Pros:

- Discreet and less noticeable under clothing.
- Suitable for physical activities, including swimming.
- Available in different absorbency levels.

Cons:

- Risk of TSS if left in for too long (more than 8 hours).
- May cause discomfort during insertion or removal, especially for first-time users.

Dr. Alyssa Dweck, a gynecologist and author of *The Complete A to Z for Your V*, advises, *"It's important to follow instructions for tampon use carefully to minimize the risk of TSS. Always choose the lowest absorbency necessary for your flow and change tampons regularly."*

3. Menstrual Cups:

- *Definition:* Menstrual cups are reusable, flexible cups made of medical-grade silicone or latex that are inserted into the vagina to collect menstrual blood. They can hold more fluid than pads or tampons and can be worn for up to 12 hours.

Pros:

- Cost-effective and environmentally friendly.
- Can be worn for longer periods.
- Reduces the risk of dryness and irritation.

Cons:

- Can be challenging to insert and remove initially.

- Requires regular cleaning and sterilization.

4. Menstrual Discs:

- *Definition:* Menstrual discs are flexible discs made of medical-grade silicone that fit at the base of the cervix to collect menstrual blood. They can be worn for up to 12 hours and are suitable for sexual activity during menstruation.

Pros:

- Can be worn during sex.
- Long-wearing and less frequent changes needed.

Cons:

- Insertion and removal can be tricky.
- Not as widely available as other products.

5. Period Underwear:

- *Definition:* Period underwear is designed with absorbent layers to capture menstrual blood. It can be worn alone or as a backup to other menstrual products.

Pros:

- Comfortable and reusable.
- Reduces waste and is eco-friendly.

Cons:

- Requires frequent washing.
- Initial cost can be higher compared to disposable products.

📢 *Call-to-Action*: Experiment with different menstrual products to find what works best for you. Consider factors such as comfort, lifestyle, menstrual flow, and environmental impact when making your choice.

4.2 Best Practices for Menstrual Hygiene

Maintaining good menstrual hygiene is vital for preventing infections and ensuring comfort. Here are some best practices:

1. Regular Changing of Menstrual Products:

- *Pads and Tampons:* Change every 4-8 hours, depending on flow.
- *Menstrual Cups and Discs*: Empty and rinse every 8-12 hours.

2. Proper Cleaning:

- *Menstrual Cups and Discs*: Rinse with mild soap and water during periods, and sterilize by boiling between cycles.
- *Period Underwear*: Rinse in cold water before machine washing.

3. Washing Hands:

- Always wash your hands before and after changing menstrual products to prevent the spread of bacteria.

4. Genital Hygiene:

- *Use Mild Soap*: Clean the external genital area with mild, unscented soap and water. Avoid douching, as it can disrupt the natural balance of bacteria in the vagina and lead to infections.

- *Wipe Correctly:* Always wipe from front to back after using the toilet to prevent the spread of bacteria from the anus to the vagina.

Dr. Sherry Ross, an obstetrician-gynecologist and author of *She-ology*, emphasizes, *"Good menstrual hygiene is about keeping yourself clean and comfortable. It's important to use products correctly and maintain regular hygiene practices to prevent infections and ensure your overall well-being."*

- 📢 Call-to-Action: Develop a consistent menstrual hygiene routine that includes regular product changes, proper cleaning, and genital hygiene. This will help you stay comfortable and healthy throughout your cycle.

4.3   Eco-Friendly Menstrual Products

With growing environmental awareness, many women are turning to eco-friendly menstrual products. These products are designed to reduce waste and have a minimal environmental impact. Here are some popular options:

1. Reusable Menstrual Cups:

- *Eco-Benefit:* Can be reused for up to 10 years, reducing waste significantly.
- *Usage:* Sterilize between cycles and clean regularly.

2. Cloth Pads:

- *Eco-Benefit:* Reusable and made from natural, biodegradable materials.
- *Usage:* Washable and can last for several years.

3. Period Underwear:

- *Eco-Benefit:* Replaces disposable products and can be reused for several years.
- *Usage:* Washable and comes in various styles and absorbencies.

4. Biodegradable Disposable Pads and Tampons:

- *Eco-Benefit*: Made from organic cotton and biodegradable materials, these products decompose faster than conventional options.
- *Usage:* Used similarly to regular disposable pads and tampons but with a lower environmental impact.
    - 📢 Call-to-Action: Consider switching to eco-friendly menstrual products. Not only do they reduce environmental impact, but they can also be cost-effective in the long run. Explore options and choose products that align with your values and lifestyle.

4.4   Innovations in Menstrual Care

The field of menstrual care is continually evolving, with new products and technologies aimed at improving comfort, convenience, and sustainability. Here are some recent innovations:

1. Smart Menstrual Products:

Smart Tampons and Pads: These products use sensors to track menstrual flow and provide data to a smartphone app, helping women understand their cycles better.

2. Self-Cleaning Menstrual Cups:

- UV Sterilization: Some menstrual cups now come with UV sterilization devices that clean and sterilize the cup, reducing the need for boiling.

3. Menstrual Tracking Apps:

- *AI and Machine Learning*: Advanced menstrual tracking apps use AI to predict periods, ovulation, and fertility windows accurately. Apps like Clue and Flo provide personalized insights and health recommendations.

4. Subscription Services:

- *Convenience:* Companies like Lola and Cora offer customizable subscription boxes that deliver organic menstrual products to your door, tailored to your cycle.

Dr. Kate White, an assistant professor of obstetrics and gynecology at Boston University, notes, *"Innovations in menstrual care are making it easier for women to manage their periods with comfort and precision. These advancements are not only improving convenience but also promoting better understanding and management of menstrual health."*

- 📣 *Call to Action*: Stay informed about new developments in menstrual care. Trying out innovative products and technologies can enhance your menstrual experience and provide valuable insights into your health.

Key Facts to Remember

✓ *Choosing Menstrual Products:* Understand the pros and cons of different menstrual products, including pads, tampons, cups, discs, and period underwear. Choose what suits your lifestyle and comfort.

✓ *Hygiene Practices*: Maintain regular menstrual hygiene by changing products frequently, cleaning reusable items properly, and practicing good genital hygiene.

✓ *Eco-Friendly Options*: Consider eco-friendly menstrual products like reusable cups, cloth pads, period underwear, and biodegradable disposables to reduce environmental impact.

✓ *Innovations:* Explore the latest innovations in menstrual care, from smart products to subscription services, to improve your menstrual health management.

By adopting good menstrual hygiene practices and exploring various product options, you can manage your menstrual cycle more effectively and comfortably. Staying informed about new developments and eco-friendly choices can further enhance your menstrual health and contribute to a sustainable future.

Chapter 5:

Nutrition and Lifestyle

Your diet and lifestyle play a crucial role in maintaining menstrual health. The foods you eat, your exercise habits, and how you manage stress can significantly impact your menstrual cycle and overall well-being. This chapter delves into the importance of a balanced diet, regular exercise, stress management, and the benefits of supplements and vitamins for menstrual health.

5.1 Diet and Menstrual Health: Foods to Embrace and Avoid

What you eat can have a profound effect on your menstrual cycle. Certain foods can help alleviate menstrual symptoms, while others can exacerbate them. Understanding the connection between diet and menstrual health is essential for managing your cycle effectively.

Foods to Embrace:

1. Leafy Greens:

- Iron-rich foods like leafy greens are crucial for preventing anemia during menstruation. Magnesium helps relax muscles and alleviate cramps.
- *Examples:* Spinach, kale, Swiss chard.

- *Benefits:* High in iron and magnesium, which can help replenish lost nutrients during menstruation and reduce muscle cramps.

2. Fruits:

- Berries and citrus fruits are rich in vitamin C, which can help with the absorption of iron and boost the immune system.
- *Examples:* Berries, oranges, apples.
- *Benefits*: Packed with vitamins and antioxidants, fruits can help reduce inflammation and provide energy.

3. Whole Grains:

- Whole grains provide sustained energy and help keep blood sugar levels stable.
- *Examples:* Oats, quinoa, brown rice.
- *Benefits*: High in fiber, which can help regulate digestion and prevent bloating.

4. Fatty Fish:

- Omega-3s have anti-inflammatory properties that can help reduce menstrual cramps.
- *Examples*: Salmon, mackerel, sardines.
- *Benefits*: Rich in omega-3 fatty acids, which can reduce inflammation and alleviate menstrual pain.

Foods to Avoid:

1. Caffeine:

- Reducing caffeine intake can help alleviate PMS symptoms like irritability and breast pain.

- *Examples*: Coffee, tea, chocolate.
- *Impact*: Can increase anxiety, irritability, and breast tenderness.

2. Salty Foods:

- High sodium intake can exacerbate bloating and water retention.
- *Examples:* Processed snacks, canned soups, fast food.
- *Impact:* Can cause water retention and bloating.

3. Sugary Foods:

- Excess sugar can contribute to inflammation and exacerbate PMS symptoms.
- *Examples*: Sweets, sodas, baked goods.
- *Impact*: Can cause blood sugar spikes and crashes, leading to mood swings and fatigue.

4. Alcohol:

- Alcohol can disrupt hormonal balance and worsen menstrual symptoms.
- *Impact:* Can interfere with hormone levels and increase menstrual discomfort.
  - 📢 *Call to Action*: Incorporate nutrient-dense foods into your diet to support menstrual health. Track how different foods affect your cycle and adjust your diet accordingly to reduce discomfort and improve overall well-being.

5.2 Exercise and Its Impact on Your Cycle

Regular physical activity is beneficial for overall health and can positively impact your menstrual cycle. Exercise helps regulate hormones, reduce stress, and alleviate menstrual symptoms. Here's how different types of exercise affect menstrual health:

1. Aerobic Exercise:

- Aerobic exercise can help reduce the severity of menstrual cramps by increasing blood flow and releasing endorphins.
- Examples: Running, swimming, cycling.
- *Benefits:* Improves cardiovascular health, increases endorphins (feel-good hormones), and reduces menstrual pain.

2. Strength Training:

- Strength training helps balance hormones and improve overall fitness, which can lead to more regular menstrual cycles.
- *Examples*: Weight lifting, resistance bands.
- *Benefits*: Builds muscle, improves metabolism, and can help regulate hormones.

3. Yoga and Pilates:

- Practicing yoga can help reduce stress and alleviate menstrual discomfort by promoting relaxation and flexibility.
- *Benefits*: Enhances flexibility, reduces stress, and can alleviate PMS symptoms.

4. Low-Impact Exercise:

- Low-impact exercises like walking can be very effective in managing menstrual symptoms and improving overall mood.
- *Examples*: Walking, tai chi.
- *Benefits*: Gentle on the body, promotes circulation, and can help reduce bloating.
  - 🔊 *Call to Action*: Incorporate regular physical activity into your routine. Aim for a mix of aerobic, strength training, and flexibility exercises to support menstrual health and overall well-being.

5.3   Stress Management for a Healthier Cycle

Stress can significantly impact your menstrual cycle, leading to irregular periods, increased PMS symptoms, and overall discomfort. Effective stress management techniques are crucial for maintaining a healthy cycle. Here are some strategies to consider:

1. Mindfulness and Meditation:

- Mindfulness meditation helps calm the mind and body, reducing the impact of stress on the menstrual cycle.
- *Benefits:* Reduces stress, improves mental clarity, and promotes relaxation.

2. Deep Breathing Exercises:

- Deep breathing exercises can help reduce stress and promote a sense of calm, which can positively affect menstrual health.

- *Benefits:* Lowers stress hormones, improves oxygen flow, and promotes relaxation.

3. Time Management:

- Effective time management can help reduce stress and create more opportunities for relaxation and self-care.
- *Benefits*: Reduces overwhelm, increases productivity, and allows for better self-care.

4. *Physical Activity:*

- Regular exercise is one of the best ways to manage stress and support menstrual health.
- *Benefits*: Reduces stress hormones, increases endorphins, and improves mood.

5. *Social Support:*

- Having a strong support network can significantly reduce stress and improve overall health.
- *Benefits:* Provides emotional support, reduces feelings of isolation, and promotes well-being.
  - 🔊 Call-to-Action: Incorporate stress management techniques into your daily routine. Experiment with mindfulness, deep breathing, exercise, time management, and social support to find what works best for you. Reducing stress can lead to a healthier menstrual cycle and improved overall well-being.

5.4 Supplements and Vitamins for Menstrual Health

Certain supplements and vitamins can help alleviate menstrual symptoms and support overall reproductive health. Here's a look at some of the most beneficial ones:

1. Magnesium:

- Magnesium is a key mineral for reducing menstrual cramps and supporting overall muscle function.
- Benefits: Reduces menstrual cramps, alleviates PMS symptoms, and supports muscle relaxation.

2. Vitamin B6:

- Vitamin B6 is crucial for mood regulation and can help reduce symptoms of PMS, including irritability and bloating.
- *Benefits*: Helps regulate mood, reduces PMS symptoms, and supports hormonal balance.

3. Omega-3 Fatty Acids:

- Omega-3 fatty acids have powerful anti-inflammatory properties that can help reduce menstrual cramps and improve overall menstrual health.
- *Sources*: Fish oil, flaxseed oil.
- *Benefits*: Reduces inflammation, alleviates menstrual pain, and supports overall health.

4. Calcium:

- Adequate calcium intake is essential for reducing PMS symptoms and supporting overall health.
- *Benefits*: Reduces PMS symptoms, supports bone health, and promotes muscle function.

5. Vitamin D:

- Vitamin D plays a crucial role in hormone regulation and can help alleviate PMS symptoms.
- Benefits: Supports hormone regulation, reduces PMS symptoms, and improves mood.

6. Herbal Supplements:

- Herbal supplements like chasteberry and evening primrose oil can be effective in managing PMS and menstrual symptoms Examples: Chasteberry, evening primrose oil.
- Benefits: Supports hormonal balance, reduces PMS symptoms, and alleviates menstrual discomfort.
  - 🔊 Call to Action: Consider incorporating supplements and vitamins into your daily routine to support menstrual health. Consult with a healthcare provider to determine the appropriate supplements for your individual needs and ensure proper dosage.

Key Facts to Remember

- ✓ Diet: Embrace nutrient-dense foods like leafy greens, fruits, whole grains, and fatty fish while avoiding caffeine, salty foods, sugary foods, and alcohol to support menstrual health.

✓ Exercise: Regular physical activity, including aerobic exercise, strength training, yoga, and low-impact exercises, can positively impact your menstrual cycle and overall well-being.

✓ Stress Management: Effective stress management techniques, such as mindfulness, deep breathing, exercise, time management, and social support, can lead to a healthier menstrual cycle.

✓ *Supplements:* Certain supplements and vitamins, including magnesium, vitamin B6, omega-3 fatty acids, calcium, vitamin D, and herbal supplements, can help alleviate menstrual symptoms and support reproductive health.

By adopting a balanced diet, maintaining regular physical activity, managing stress effectively, and incorporating beneficial supplements, you can support your menstrual health and overall well-being. These lifestyle changes can help you manage menstrual symptoms more effectively and improve your quality of life.

Chapter 6:

Emotional Well-Being

Understanding and managing emotional well-being is a crucial aspect of menstrual health. Hormonal fluctuations throughout the menstrual cycle can significantly impact your mood, mental health, and overall emotional state. This chapter explores mood swings and emotional changes, the role of mindfulness, the importance of building a support system, and the benefits of journaling and self-reflection. By adopting effective strategies, you can better navigate the emotional ups and downs associated with your cycle.

6.1   Mood Swings and Emotional Changes

Hormonal changes during the menstrual cycle can lead to mood swings and emotional fluctuations. These changes are a normal part of the menstrual cycle but can be challenging to manage.

Understanding Hormonal Influences:

- **Estrogen:** This hormone rises during the first half of the menstrual cycle (the follicular phase), peaking just before ovulation. High levels of estrogen can boost mood and energy levels.

- ***Progesterone:*** After ovulation, progesterone levels increase during the second half of the cycle (the luteal phase). Elevated progesterone can cause moodiness, irritability, and fatigue.
- ***Serotonin:*** This neurotransmitter, often referred to as the "feel-good" chemical, can fluctuate with hormone levels, impacting mood. Lower serotonin levels can lead to feelings of sadness or depression.

Expert Advice: Dr. Christiane Northrup, a women's health expert, explains, *"Understanding the natural rhythm of your menstrual cycle can help you anticipate emotional changes and take proactive steps to manage them."*

Strategies for Managing Mood Swings:

1. Maintain a Balanced Diet:
- Eating a diet rich in whole grains, lean proteins, healthy fats, and plenty of fruits and vegetables can stabilize blood sugar levels and improve mood.
- Avoiding excessive sugar and caffeine can help reduce mood swings.

2. Regular Exercise:
- Physical activity releases endorphins, which are natural mood lifters.
- Activities like walking, running, yoga, and dancing can help alleviate stress and improve mood.

3. Sleep Well:
- Getting enough sleep is crucial for emotional well-being.
- Aim for 7-9 hours of quality sleep per night.

4. Practice Relaxation Techniques:

- Techniques such as deep breathing, meditation, and progressive muscle relaxation can help manage stress and emotional fluctuations.
  - 🔊 Call to Action: Pay attention to how your mood changes throughout your menstrual cycle. Keep a mood diary to track patterns and identify effective coping strategies that work for you.

6.2 Mindfulness and Mental Health During Your Cycle

Mindfulness is a powerful tool for managing emotional health, particularly during the menstrual cycle. It involves being fully present in the moment and accepting your thoughts and feelings without judgment.

Benefits of Mindfulness:

- Reduces Stress: Mindfulness can lower cortisol levels, reducing stress and anxiety.
- Improves Emotional Regulation: Helps you become more aware of your emotional triggers and responses.
- Enhances Self-Awareness: Promotes a deeper understanding of your emotional and physical states.

Mindfulness Techniques:

1. Meditation:

- Practice: Set aside a few minutes each day to sit quietly, focus on your breath, and observe your thoughts. Start with short sessions and gradually increasing the duration as you become more comfortable.

2. Body Scan:

- Body scans can help you become more in tune with your body and identify areas of tension or discomfort.
- *Practice:* Lie down in a comfortable position and focus on each part of your body, starting from your toes and moving up to your head. Notice any sensations or tension.

3. Mindful Breathing:

- *Practice*: Take slow, deep breaths, focusing on the sensation of the breath entering and leaving your body.
- *Expert Advice:* Dr. Andrew Weil, a holistic health expert, suggests practicing 4-7-8 breathing (inhale for 4 seconds, hold for 7 seconds, exhale for 8 seconds) to promote relaxation.

4. Mindful Movement:

- Mindful movement combines physical exercise with mental focus, enhancing both physical and emotional well-being.
- *Practice:* Engage in activities like yoga, tai chi, or walking with a focus on the movements and sensations of your body.
  - 🔊 *Call to Action:* Incorporate mindfulness practices into your daily routine. Start with simple exercises like mindful breathing or a body scan and gradually explore other techniques. Mindfulness can help you manage

emotional changes more effectively and improve your overall mental health.

6.3   Building a Support System

Having a strong support system is vital for emotional well-being, especially during challenging times in your menstrual cycle. Support from family, friends, and communities can provide comfort, advice, and understanding.

Types of Support Systems:

1. Family and Friends:
- Importance of maintaining strong relationships cannot be overemphasized. Healthy relationships are key to emotional well-being. Make time to connect with loved ones regularly.
- *Benefits*: Offer emotional support, practical help, and a listening ear.

2. Support Groups:
- *Benefits:* Provide a safe space to share experiences and gain insights from others who understand what you're going through. Sharing your story with others can be incredibly healing. It helps you realize you're not alone.

3. Therapists and Counselors:
- Therapy can provide valuable tools for managing emotional health and improving quality of life.
- *Benefits:* Offer professional guidance and coping strategies for managing emotional challenges.

4. Online Communities:

- Online communities can be a great resource for support and information, but it's important to choose reputable and positive groups.
- *Benefits:* Offer convenience and anonymity, providing access to a broad range of perspectives and advice.
  - 🔊 *Call to Action*: Identify and build your support network. Reach out to family and friends, join support groups, consider therapy if needed, and explore online communities. Having a strong support system can significantly improve your emotional well-being.

6.4　Journaling and Self-Reflection

Journaling is a powerful tool for self-reflection and emotional health. It allows you to process your thoughts and feelings, track patterns, and gain insights into your emotional state.

Benefits of Journaling:

- *Clarifies Thoughts and Feelings:* Writing helps you understand and articulate your emotions.
- *Reduces Stress:* Journaling can be a cathartic release, helping to reduce anxiety and stress.
- *Tracks Patterns*: Keeping a journal can help you identify emotional patterns related to your menstrual cycle.
- *Encourages Self-Reflection:* Promotes personal growth and self-awareness.

Types of Journaling:

1. Daily Journaling:

- *Practice:* Spend a few minutes each day writing about your thoughts, feelings, and experiences.

2. Gratitude Journaling:

- *Practice:* Write about things you are grateful for each day. Practicing gratitude can improve emotional well-being and increase resilience.

3. Emotion Tracking:

- *Practice:* Note your emotions throughout the day and any triggers or patterns you observe. Tracking your emotions can help you identify triggers and develop coping strategies.

4. Reflective Journaling:

- *Practice:* Reflect on significant events, decisions, and experiences, and analyze your responses. Reflective journaling can lead to profound insights and personal growth.
  - *Call to Action:* Start a journaling practice that suits your lifestyle. Whether it's daily writing, gratitude lists, or emotion tracking, journaling can help you process emotions, reduce stress, and gain self-awareness.

Key Facts to Remember

✓ *Mood Swings and Emotional Changes*: Hormonal fluctuations during your menstrual cycle can cause mood swings. Managing diet, exercise, sleep, and relaxation techniques can help stabilize mood.

✓ *Mindfulness:* Practicing mindfulness through meditation, deep breathing, body scans, and mindful movement can reduce stress and improve emotional regulation.

✓ *Support System:* Building a strong support system with family, friends, support groups, therapists, and online communities is essential for emotional well-being.

✓ *Journaling:* Journaling helps clarify thoughts and feelings, reduce stress, track emotional patterns, and promote self-reflection and personal growth.

By understanding and managing your emotional well-being through these strategies, you can navigate the emotional challenges of your menstrual cycle more effectively. Embrace these practices to enhance your overall mental health and well-being.

Chapter 7:

Special Considerations

Menstrual health is a dynamic aspect of a woman's life that changes through different life stages and can be affected by various health conditions. Understanding these special considerations is vital for managing your menstrual health effectively. This chapter covers menstrual health in adolescents, changes during pregnancy and postpartum, what to expect during perimenopause and menopause, and managing menstrual health with chronic conditions.

7.1   Menstrual Health in Adolescents

Adolescence marks the beginning of menstruation, known as menarche, typically occurring between ages 10 and 15. This phase involves significant hormonal changes and can be both exciting and challenging for young girls.

Understanding Menarche:

- *Menarche*: The first menstrual period signifies the onset of reproductive capability.
- *Hormonal Changes:* The hypothalamus signals the pituitary gland to release hormones (FSH and LH) that stimulate the

ovaries to produce estrogen and progesterone, initiating menstrual cycles.

Managing Adolescent Menstrual Health:

It's essential to provide adolescents with accurate information about their bodies to promote a healthy and positive attitude towards menstruation.

1. Education and Communication:

- It is important to educate young girls about menstruation, including what to expect, how to manage periods, and the significance of menstrual health. Open communication with a trusted adult can alleviate anxiety and build confidence.

2. Healthy Lifestyle:

- *Diet:* Encourage a balanced diet rich in iron, calcium, and vitamins to support overall health.
- *Exercise:* Promote regular physical activity to improve mood and reduce menstrual discomfort.

3. Menstrual Hygiene:

- *Products:* Parents of adolescent should introduce various menstrual products such as (pads, tampons, cups) to their girls and guide them on proper usage.
- *Hygiene Practices*: Emphasize the importance of regular changing and proper disposal of menstrual products to prevent infections.

4. Emotional Support:

- *Peer Support:* Encourage participation in support groups or discussions with peers to share experiences.
- *Parental Involvement:* Parents should provide emotional support and understanding during this transition.
  - 🔊 *Call to Action:* Parents and guardians should create an open and supportive environment for adolescents to discuss menstrual health. Providing education, resources, and emotional support is crucial for building a positive and informed approach to menstruation.

7.2 Menstrual Changes During Pregnancy and Postpartum

Pregnancy and postpartum periods bring significant hormonal and physical changes that impact menstruation.

1. Menstrual Changes During Pregnancy:

- *Cessation of Menstruation:* Menstruation stops during pregnancy due to elevated levels of hormones like human chorionic gonadotropin (hCG), progesterone, and estrogen, which maintain the pregnancy.
- *Spotting:* Light spotting can occur in early pregnancy, often due to implantation bleeding.

2. Postpartum Menstrual Changes:

- *Lochia:* Postpartum bleeding known as lochia occurs for 4-6 weeks after childbirth. It starts heavy and gradually lightens.

- *Resumption of Menstruation:* The return of regular menstrual cycles varies. Breastfeeding mothers may experience a delay in the return of periods due to the hormone prolactin, which suppresses ovulation.

Expert Advice: Dr. Mary Jane Minkin, a gynecologist, explains, *"Postpartum menstrual changes are highly individual. Women should monitor their bodies and consult healthcare providers if they have concerns."*

Managing Postpartum Menstrual Health:

1. Monitor Bleeding:

- *Lochia:* Track the color and amount of postpartum bleeding. Seek medical advice if you experience heavy bleeding or large clots.
- *Menstruation*: Observe the return of regular periods and any changes in cycle length or flow.

2. Postpartum Care:

- Nutrition: Eat a balanced diet rich in iron and vitamins to support recovery and lactation.
- *Rest:* Ensure adequate rest to aid healing and manage stress.

3. Breastfeeding:

- *Impact on Menstruation:* Understand that exclusive breastfeeding may delay the return of periods.
- *Contraception:* Discuss postpartum contraception options with your healthcare provider to avoid unintended pregnancy.

🔊 *Call to Action:* Postpartum women should maintain regular check-ups with their healthcare provider, track menstrual changes, and seek medical advice if they experience abnormal bleeding or other concerns.

7.3 Perimenopause and Menopause: What to Expect

Perimenopause and menopause mark the end of reproductive years and bring significant hormonal changes affecting menstrual health.

Understanding Perimenopause and Menopause:

- *Perimenopause:* The transition period leading up to menopause, characterized by fluctuating hormone levels and irregular menstrual cycles. It can last 4-10 years.
- *Menopause:* Defined as the cessation of menstruation for 12 consecutive months, typically occurring around age 51. Hormone levels decline, ending reproductive capability.

Common Symptoms:

- *Irregular Periods:* Cycles may become longer or shorter, with varying flow intensity.
- *Hot Flashes:* Sudden feelings of warmth, often accompanied by sweating.
- *Night Sweats:* Hot flashes occurring during sleep, causing night-time sweating.
- *Mood Changes*: Increased risk of mood swings, anxiety, and depression.

- *Vaginal Dryness:* Decreased estrogen levels can lead to vaginal dryness and discomfort.

Expert Advice: Dr. JoAnn Manson, a menopause expert, advises, *"Understanding the changes occurring during perimenopause and menopause can help women manage symptoms and maintain quality of life."*

Managing Menopausal Symptoms:

1. Lifestyle Modifications:

- *Diet:* Consume a diet rich in phytoestrogens (soy, flaxseed) and calcium to support bone health.
- *Exercise*: Engage in regular physical activity to improve mood, maintain weight, and strengthen bones.

2. Hormone Therapy:

- *Options*: Discuss hormone replacement therapy (HRT) with your healthcare provider to manage severe symptoms.
- *Risks and Benefits*: Understand the potential risks and benefits of HRT to make an informed decision.

3. Non-Hormonal Treatments:

- *Medications*: Consider non-hormonal medications for hot flashes and mood stabilization.
- *Natural Remedies*: Explore natural remedies like black cohosh or evening primrose oil, but consult your healthcare provider first.

4. Emotional Support:

- *Support Groups*: Join menopause support groups to share experiences and gain insights.
- *Counseling*: Seek professional counseling if experiencing significant mood changes or emotional distress.
  - 🔊 *Call-to-Action:* Women approaching perimenopause and menopause should educate themselves about the changes occurring during this phase. Regular consultations with healthcare providers can help manage symptoms and maintain overall health.

7.4 Managing Menstrual Health with Chronic Conditions

Chronic conditions can significantly impact menstrual health. Understanding the interplay between chronic illnesses and menstruation is crucial for effective management.

Common Chronic Conditions Affecting Menstrual Health:

1. Polycystic Ovary Syndrome (PCOS):

- *Symptoms*: Irregular periods, excessive hair growth, acne, and weight gain.
- *Management*: Lifestyle changes, medications to regulate periods, and treatment for insulin resistance.

2. Endometriosis:

- *Symptoms*: Painful periods, heavy bleeding, and infertility.
- *Management:* Pain relief medications, hormonal treatments, and surgical options for severe cases.

3. Diabetes:

- *Impact:* Uncontrolled blood sugar levels can lead to irregular periods and exacerbated menstrual symptoms.
- *Management:* Blood sugar control through diet, exercise, and medications.

4. Thyroid Disorders:

- *Impact:* Hypothyroidism or hyperthyroidism can cause irregular periods and other menstrual disturbances.
- *Management:* Thyroid hormone replacement or medications to regulate thyroid function.

5. Autoimmune Conditions:

- *Examples:* Lupus, rheumatoid arthritis.
- *Impact:* Medications and the condition itself can affect menstrual cycles.
- *Management:* Close monitoring and coordination with healthcare providers. Managing chronic conditions effectively is crucial for maintaining regular menstrual cycles and overall reproductive health.

Strategies for Managing Menstrual Health with Chronic Conditions:

1. Regular Monitoring:

- *Track Symptoms:* Keep a detailed record of menstrual symptoms and any correlations with your chronic condition.

- *Medical Check-Ups:* Schedule regular check-ups with your healthcare provider to monitor both menstrual health and the chronic condition.

2. Medications and Treatments:

- *Adherence:* Follow prescribed treatment plans and medications to manage chronic conditions effectively.
- *Adjustments*: Work with your healthcare provider to adjust treatments as needed to minimize menstrual disruptions.

3. Lifestyle Modifications:

- *Diet and Exercise*: Maintain a healthy diet and regular exercise routine to support overall health and menstrual regularity.
- *Stress Management*: Implement stress-reduction techniques like mindfulness, yoga, and relaxation exercises.

4. Communication with Healthcare Providers:

- *Inform Providers:* Ensure all healthcare providers are aware of your chronic condition and its impact on menstrual health.
- *Integrated Care*: Seek coordinated care approaches that address both the chronic condition and menstrual health.
  - 🔊 *Call to Action:* Women with chronic conditions should work closely with their healthcare providers to manage their health comprehensively. Keeping detailed records, adhering to treatment plans, and making lifestyle adjustments can help maintain regular menstrual cycles and overall well-being.

Key Facts to Remember

✓ *Adolescents*: Educate young girls about menstrual health, promote healthy lifestyles, and provide emotional support.

✓ *Pregnancy and Postpartum*: Understand menstrual changes during pregnancy and postpartum, monitor bleeding, and maintain postpartum care.

✓ *Perimenopause and Menopause*: Recognize the symptoms and manage them through lifestyle changes, hormone therapy, and emotional support.

✓ *Chronic Conditions:* Manage menstrual health by monitoring symptoms, adhering to treatment plans, and maintaining communication with healthcare providers.

By understanding these special considerations and implementing effective strategies, women can better manage their menstrual health throughout different life stages and health conditions.

Chapter 8:

BREAKING THE STIGMA

Menstruation is a natural biological process, yet it has been surrounded by stigma and taboo across various cultures and societies. This chapter delves into cultural perspectives on menstruation, the importance of advocating for menstrual health awareness, effective ways to talk to teens about menstrual health, and strategies for creating inclusive environments in work and school settings.

8.1   Cultural Perspectives on Menstruation

Menstrual stigma has deep roots in cultural beliefs and traditions. Understanding these perspectives is crucial for breaking the cycle of silence and misinformation.

Historical and Cultural Context:

Cultural perceptions of menstruation shape how women experience their periods and influence public policies and health practices. These cultural perceptions include:

- *Taboos and Myths:* Many cultures have myths that portray menstruation as impure or shameful. For instance, in some parts of India, menstruating women are not allowed to enter temples or kitchens.

- *Rituals and Practices:* Some cultures have specific rituals for menstruating women. In Nepal, the practice of "Chhaupadi" involves isolating women in small huts during their menstrual period.

Impact of Cultural Perspectives:

- *Health and Hygiene*: Stigmatization can lead to inadequate access to menstrual hygiene products and facilities, impacting women's health.
- *Education:* Girls often miss school during their periods due to stigma and lack of resources, affecting their education and future opportunities.
- *Psychological Well-Being*: Negative cultural attitudes can lead to feelings of shame and embarrassment, affecting mental health.

Strategies for Change:

1. Education and Awareness:

- *Promote Education*: Educate communities about the biological facts of menstruation to dispel myths and taboos. Education is the key to transforming societal attitudes towards menstruation.

2. Empowerment Initiatives:

- *Support Groups:* Create safe spaces where women can share experiences and support each other.
- *Community Programs*: Implement community-based programs that encourage open discussions about menstruation.

3. Policy Changes:

- *Advocate for Policies*: Support policies that provide free or subsidized menstrual products and promote menstrual health education.
- *Global Efforts*: Organizations like UNICEF and WHO work globally to improve menstrual health and break stigmas.
  - ◀» *Call-to-Action:* Engage in conversations about menstruation in your community. Advocate for educational programs and policies that promote menstrual health awareness and combat stigma.

8.2   Advocating for Menstrual Health Awareness

Advocacy plays a crucial role in raising awareness about menstrual health and challenging societal norms that perpetuate stigma. Advocacy is about creating a movement that not only addresses immediate needs but also builds long-term cultural change.

Why Advocacy Matters:

- *Awareness and Education*: Advocacy helps spread accurate information about menstruation, dispelling myths and fostering a more informed society.
- *Policy and Infrastructure*: Effective advocacy can lead to better policies and improved infrastructure for menstrual health, such as providing free menstrual products in schools and public places.
- *Empowerment:* Advocacy empowers women and girls by normalizing conversations about menstruation and

encouraging them to take control of their menstrual health.

Ways to Advocate:

1. Public Campaigns:

- *Social media:* Use platforms like Instagram, Twitter, and Facebook to spread awareness and share information.
- *Events and Workshops*: Organize events and workshops to educate the public and engage in discussions about menstrual health.

2. Collaborations:

- *Partner with NGOs*: Work with non-governmental organizations that focus on menstrual health and hygiene.
- *School Programs*: Collaborate with schools to implement menstrual health education programs.

3. Policy Advocacy:

- *Lobby for Change:* Advocate for laws and policies that support menstrual health, such as tax exemptions for menstrual products.
- *Grassroots Movements:* Encourage grassroots movements to push for local changes and community-based solutions.

4. Storytelling:

- *Personal Narratives*: Share personal stories about menstrual experiences to humanize the issue and foster empathy.

- *Media Engagement*: Use media outlets to highlight menstrual health issues and advocate for change.
- 🔊 *Call-to-Action:* Get involved in menstrual health advocacy by joining or supporting organizations dedicated to this cause. Use your voice to raise awareness and push for policy changes that improve menstrual health and hygiene.

8.3 Talking to Teens About Menstrual Health

Educating teens about menstrual health is essential for their physical, emotional, and psychological well-being. Creating an open and supportive environment for these conversations can empower teens to understand and manage their menstrual health effectively.

Why It's Important:

Parents and educators should approach conversations about menstruation with openness and positivity to encourage trust and understanding. These should include:

- *Early Education*: Providing accurate information early helps demystify menstruation and build confidence.
- *Health and Hygiene*: Educating teens about menstrual hygiene practices prevents health issues and promotes well-being.
- *Emotional Support:* Open conversations help teens feel supported and reduce feelings of embarrassment or shame.

Tips for Talking to Teens:

1. Start Early:

- *Age-Appropriate Information*: Begin discussions about body changes and menstruation before puberty, using age-appropriate language.
- *Normalize the Conversation*: Integrate menstrual health into regular health education to normalize it.

2. Be Open and Honest:

- *Factual Information*: Provide accurate and comprehensive information about the menstrual cycle and related topics.
- *Encourage Questions*: Create a safe space for teens to ask questions without fear of judgment.

3. Use Educational Resources:

- *Books and Websites:* Utilize books, websites, and other educational materials designed for teens.
- *Workshops and Programs*: Participate in or organize educational workshops and programs on menstrual health.

4. Address Emotional Aspects:

- *Support and Empathy:* Offer emotional support and validate their feelings about menstruation.
- *Positive Attitude*: Encourage a positive attitude towards menstruation as a normal and healthy part of life.
  - 🔊 *Call-to-Action:* Parents, guardians, and educators should prioritize menstrual health education for teens.

Use available resources and create an open dialogue to ensure teens feel informed and supported.

8.4 Creating Inclusive Work and School Environments

Creating inclusive environments in work and school settings is essential for supporting menstrual health and breaking the stigma associated with menstruation.

Why Inclusivity Matters:

Inclusive environments that address menstrual health needs are fundamental to achieving gender equity in education and the workplace. The impact include:

- *Health and Comfort:* Inclusive environments ensure that individuals have access to necessary menstrual products and facilities, promoting health and comfort.
- *Productivity and Participation:* When menstrual health needs are met, individuals can participate fully in work and school activities without disruptions.
- *Diversity and Equity:* Addressing menstrual health in policies and practices promotes gender equity and supports diversity.

Strategies for Creating Inclusivity:

1. Access to Menstrual Products:

- *Free Products:* Provide free menstrual products in restrooms at schools and workplaces.

- *Dispensers:* Install dispensers for pads and tampons in accessible locations.

2. Facilities and Accommodations:

- *Private Spaces*: Ensure there are private and clean facilities for changing menstrual products.
- *Flexible Policies*: Implement flexible policies that allow for menstrual leave or breaks if needed.

3. Education and Training:

- *Awareness Programs*: Conduct awareness programs to educate staff and students about menstrual health and inclusivity.
- *Training:* Train educators, managers, and HR personnel on menstrual health and how to support individuals.

4. Supportive Culture:

- *Open Dialogue*: Foster a culture of openness where discussing menstrual health is normalized and stigma-free.
- *Policy Integration:* Integrate menstrual health considerations into broader health and wellness policies.
  - 🔊 *Call-to-Action*: Advocate for and implement inclusive policies and practices in your school or workplace. Ensure that menstrual health needs are addressed to create supportive and equitable environments.

Key Facts to Remember

✓ *Cultural Perspectives*: Cultural beliefs and practices significantly influence how menstruation is perceived and managed. Education and community programs can help dispel myths and reduce stigma.

✓ *Advocacy:* Effective advocacy raises awareness, promotes policy changes, and empowers individuals to speak openly about menstrual health.

✓ *Teen Education:* Early and open communication about menstrual health is crucial for teens' physical and emotional well-being. Use educational resources and encourage questions.

✓ *Inclusivily*: Inclusive environments in work and school settings support menstrual health, promote equity, and enhance participation and productivity. Implement policies and provide access to menstrual products and facilities.

By understanding these aspects and taking proactive steps, we can break the stigma surrounding menstruation and create a more informed, supportive, and equitable society.

Chapter 9:

Resources and Support

Navigating menstrual health can be a complex journey, but with the right resources and support, it becomes manageable and empowering. This chapter provides guidance on finding the right healthcare provider, joining support groups and online communities, exploring recommended reading and educational materials, and using apps and tools for menstrual health.

9.1   Finding the Right Healthcare Provider

Choosing a healthcare provider who understands and respects your menstrual health needs is crucial for effective management and support.

Why It Matters:

- *Specialized Knowledge*: Healthcare providers with expertise in gynecology and reproductive health can offer accurate diagnoses and personalized treatment plans.
- *Comfort and Trust*: Building a trusting relationship with your provider ensures open communication and better health outcomes.

- *Comprehensive Care*: A good provider will consider all aspects of your health, including physical, emotional, and mental well-being.

Expert Advice: Dr. Lisa Masterson, an OB-GYN and women's health advocate, emphasizes, *"Finding a healthcare provider who listens and understands your needs is the cornerstone of effective menstrual health management."*

Steps to Find the Right Provider:

1. Research and Referrals:

- *Ask for Recommendations*: Seek recommendations from friends, family, or your primary care physician.
- *Online Reviews*: Look at online reviews and ratings to gauge patient satisfaction.

2. Check Credentials and Experience:

- *Board Certification*: Ensure the provider is board-certified in gynecology or reproductive health.
- *Special Interests:* Find out if they have experience in specific areas of menstrual health, such as endometriosis or PCOS.

3. Initial Consultation:

- *Comfort Level*: Assess how comfortable you feel discussing your menstrual health with the provider.
- *Communication Style*: Consider whether the provider communicates clearly and answers your questions thoroughly.

4. Practical Considerations:

- *Location and Availability*: Ensure the provider's office is conveniently located and their availability aligns with your schedule.
- *Insurance and Costs*: Verify that the provider accepts your insurance and discuss potential costs.
  - 📢 *Call to Action*: Take the time to find a healthcare provider who meets your needs and makes you feel comfortable. Don't hesitate to switch providers if you're not satisfied with the care you're receiving.

9.2   Support Groups and Online Communities

Connecting with others who share similar experiences can provide emotional support, practical advice, and a sense of community.

Benefits of Support Groups and Online Communities:

- *Shared Experiences*: Hearing others' stories can validate your experiences and make you feel less alone.
- *Practical Advice*: Gain practical tips and strategies for managing menstrual symptoms and improving your quality of life.
- *Emotional Support*: Receive empathy and encouragement from people who understand what you're going through.

Expert Advice: Dr. Jen Gunter, a gynecologist and author, says, *"Support groups can be incredibly beneficial for emotional well-being and can provide practical insights that you might not get from a clinical setting."*

Types of Support Available:

1. In-Person Support Groups:

- *Local Health Centers*: Many health centers and hospitals offer support groups for menstrual health conditions like endometriosis and PCOS.
- *Community Organizations*: Look for community organizations that focus on women's health and wellness.

2. Online Communities:

- *Social Media*: Platforms like Facebook and Reddit have groups dedicated to menstrual health topics.
- *Specialized Forums*: Websites like *MyEndometriosisTeam* and *SoulCysters* offer forums for specific conditions.

3. Professional-Led Groups:

- *Therapist-Led*: Some support groups are led by mental health professionals who can provide structured guidance.
- *Healthcare-Led*: Healthcare providers may host groups to discuss medical management and treatment options.
  - 🔊 *Call to Action*: Join a support group or online community to connect with others, share experiences, and gain support. Participation can enhance your understanding of menstrual health and provide valuable resources.

9.3   Recommended Reading and Educational Materials

Books, articles, and educational materials can deepen your understanding of menstrual health and provide reliable information.

Why Reading Matters:

- *Informed Decisions*: Knowledge empowers you to make informed decisions about your health.
- *Comprehensive Understanding*: Educational materials can offer a broader perspective on menstrual health, covering various topics and conditions.
- *Continual Learning*: Staying updated with the latest research and information helps you manage your health more effectively.
  - 📢 *Expert Advice:* Dr. Christiane Northrup, author of "Women's Bodies, Women's Wisdom," suggests, *"Investing time in learning about your body and menstrual health can profoundly impact your overall well-being."*

Recommended Books and Articles:

1. Books:

- *"The Vagina Bible"* by Dr. Jen Gunter: A comprehensive guide to women's health, including menstrual health.
- *"Period Repair Manual"* by Lara Briden: A practical guide to treating period problems with natural treatments.
- *"In the Flo"* by Alisa Vitti: A book on syncing with your menstrual cycle for better health and productivity.

2. Articles and Journals:

- *PubMed and ResearchGate*: Access scientific studies and journal articles on menstrual health topics.
- *Online Magazines*: Websites like Healthline, WebMD, and Mayo Clinic offer articles on menstrual health.

3. Educational Websites:

- *Menstrual Health Hub*: Provides resources and information on menstrual health education.
- *Planned Parenthood*: Offers educational materials and resources on menstrual health and reproductive care.
  - 🔊 *Call to Action*: Explore the recommended reading materials to enhance your knowledge of menstrual health. Make a habit of staying informed about the latest research and developments in the field.

9.4   Apps and Tools for Menstrual Health

Technology can play a significant role in managing menstrual health by providing tools for tracking cycles, symptoms, and health data.

Benefits of Using Apps and Tools:

- *Cycle Tracking*: Monitor your menstrual cycle, including start and end dates, flow intensity, and symptoms.
- *Health Insights*: Gain insights into patterns and trends in your cycle, helping you predict periods and ovulation.
- *Personalized Reminders:* Set reminders for medication, appointments, and other health-related tasks.
- *Data Sharing:* Share your data with healthcare providers for more informed consultations.
  - 🔊 *Expert Advice*: Dr. Tania Adib, a consultant gynecologist, notes, *"Menstrual health apps can be invaluable for tracking cycles and symptoms, providing both convenience and crucial health insights."*

Popular Menstrual Health Apps:

1. Clue:

- *Features*: Tracks periods, ovulation, and symptoms; provides cycle predictions and health insights.
- *User-Friendly:* Simple interface and customizable tracking options.

2. Flo:

- *Features*: Period tracker, ovulation calculator, health insights, and personalized health plans.

- *Community Support*: Access to a community of users and expert advice.

3. Period Tracker by GP Apps:

- *Features:* Tracks menstrual cycles, symptoms, moods, and more.
- *Privacy*: Offers strong privacy settings to protect user data.

4. MyFLO:

- *Features:* Tracks menstrual cycles and symptoms, provides recommendations for diet and exercise based on cycle phase.
- *Holistic Approach*: Integrates a holistic approach to menstrual health management.

5. Ovia Health:

- *Features*: Comprehensive health tracker for periods, fertility, and pregnancy.
- *Customizable*: Allows for extensive personalization of tracking categories.
  - 🔊 *Call to Action*: Download and use a menstrual health app that fits your needs. Regular tracking can provide valuable insights into your menstrual cycle and overall health, aiding in effective management and communication with your healthcare provider.

Key Facts to Remember

✓ *Healthcare Providers*: Finding the right healthcare provider is crucial for effective menstrual health management. Ensure your provider is experienced, communicative, and trustworthy.

✓ *Support Groups*: Support groups and online communities offer emotional support, practical advice, and a sense of belonging. Join a group to connect with others and share experiences.

✓ *Educational Materials:* Reading books, articles, and educational materials enhances your understanding of menstrual health and empowers you to make informed decisions.

✓ *Apps and Tools:* Utilize menstrual health apps to track your cycle, monitor symptoms, and gain health insights. These tools can improve self-management and facilitate better healthcare interactions.

By leveraging these resources and support systems, you can take charge of your menstrual health, stay informed, and build a supportive network that enhances your overall well-being.

Chapter 10:

YOUR MENSTRUAL HEALTH JOURNEY

Embarking on your menstrual health journey is a deeply personal and empowering process. This chapter guides you through creating a personalized menstrual health plan, setting achievable goals, reflecting on your progress, and staying informed and empowered for the future.

10.1   Creating a Personal Menstrual Health Plan

A personalized menstrual health plan helps you take control of your health and manage your menstrual cycle effectively.

Steps to Create Your Plan:

A personalized menstrual health plan empowers women to take control of their health and make informed decisions about their bodies.

1. Understand Your Cycle:

- *Track Your Cycle*: Use a menstrual health app or a calendar to track your period start and end dates, flow intensity, and symptoms. This helps you identify patterns and predict future cycles.
- *Identify Symptoms*: Note any symptoms you experience, such as cramps, bloating, mood swings, or fatigue.

Understanding your symptoms can help you manage them better.

2. *Consult a Healthcare Provider*:

- *Professional Guidance:* Schedule a consultation with a gynecologist or healthcare provider to discuss your menstrual health. They can provide insights based on your tracking data and suggest appropriate treatments or lifestyle changes.
- *Regular Check-Ups:* Regular check-ups ensure that any potential issues are identified and addressed early.

3. *Set Health Goals:*

- *Specific Goals*: Define specific, measurable, achievable, relevant, and time-bound (SMART) goals for your menstrual health. For example, you might aim to reduce menstrual cramps by incorporating regular exercise and hydration.
- *Holistic Approach:* Consider all aspects of your health, including diet, exercise, stress management, and mental well-being.

4. *Choose Management Strategies:*

- *Diet and Nutrition:* Incorporate foods rich in vitamins and minerals that support menstrual health, such as leafy greens, nuts, and seeds.
- *Exercise*: Regular physical activity can help reduce symptoms like cramps and improve overall health.
- *Stress Management:* Practice stress-reducing activities like yoga, meditation, or deep breathing exercises.

5. Implement and Adjust:

- *Consistency:* Stick to your plan consistently, making adjustments as needed based on your symptoms and health goals.
- *Monitor Progress:* Regularly review your tracking data and health goals to assess your progress and make necessary changes.
  - 🔊 *Call-to-Action*: Start creating your menstrual health plan today. Track your cycle, consult with a healthcare provider, set specific goals, and choose strategies that work for you.

10.2   Setting Goals for Better Menstrual Health

Setting goals helps you focus on specific areas of improvement and track your progress over time.

Why Goal Setting is Important:

Setting goals transforms a vision of something you desire into a reality. The following are required for effective goal setting:

- *Focus and Direction*: Goals provide a clear direction and help you focus on what matters most for your menstrual health.
- *Motivation:* Achieving small milestones can boost your motivation and encourage you to stay committed to your health plan.
- *Measurable Progress*: Goals allow you to measure your progress and make adjustments as needed.

Steps to Set Effective Goals:

1. Identify Areas for Improvement:

- *Symptom Management:* Focus on reducing specific symptoms like cramps, heavy bleeding, or mood swings.
- *Lifestyle Changes*: Set goals related to diet, exercise, and stress management.

2. Define SMART Goals:

- *Specific:* Clearly define what you want to achieve. For example, "I want to reduce my menstrual cramps."
- *Measurable*: Set criteria to measure your progress. "I will track my pain levels daily."
- *Achievable*: Ensure your goal is realistic. "I will incorporate 30 minutes of exercise three times a week."
- *Relevant*: Align your goal with your overall health objectives. "Exercise can help reduce cramps."
- *Time-Bound*: Set a timeframe for achieving your goal. "I aim to see improvements in three months."

3. Create an Action Plan:

- *Steps to Achieve*: Outline the steps you need to take to reach your goal. For example, "Join a gym, start a yoga class, and track exercise sessions."
- *Resources Needed*: Identify any resources you need, such as a fitness app, a nutrition guide, or support from a healthcare provider.

4. Monitor and Adjust:

- *Regular Review:* Regularly review your progress and make adjustments as needed.
- *Celebrate Achievements*: Celebrate small victories to stay motivated.
  - 📣 Call-to-Action: Set your menstrual health goals today. Define what you want to achieve, create an action plan, and start working towards better menstrual health.

10.3   Reflecting on Your Progress

Reflecting on your progress is essential for understanding what works, what needs adjustment, and celebrating your achievements. Reflection is a powerful tool for personal growth and understanding. It allows you to learn from your experiences and improve continuously.

Why Reflection Matters:

- o *Self-Awareness*: Reflection helps you become more aware of your body's responses to different strategies.
- o *Learning and Growth*: It provides insights into what works best for you, promoting continuous learning and improvement.
- o *Motivation:* Recognizing your progress boosts motivation *and* confidence.

Steps to Reflect Effectively:

1. Regular Check-Ins:

Monthly Review: At the end of each cycle, review your tracking data, symptoms, and health goals. Note any patterns or changes.

Journal: Keep a menstrual health journal to document your experiences, thoughts, and reflections.

2. Evaluate Strategies:

What Worked: Identify strategies that helped reduce symptoms or improve your overall well-being.

Challenges: Note any challenges or obstacles you faced and consider how to address them.

3. Adjust Goals and Plans:

Refine Goals: Based on your reflections, refine your goals to better align with your needs and progress.

Adapt Strategies: Adjust your health plan to include more effective strategies or remove those that aren't working.

4. Seek Feedback:

Healthcare Provider: Share your reflections with your healthcare provider for professional insights and advice.

Support Group: Discuss your experiences with a support group to gain different perspectives and suggestions.

🔊 *Call-to-Action*: Make reflection a regular part of your menstrual health journey. Set aside time each month to review your progress, adjust your plans, and celebrate your achievements.

10.4 Looking Ahead: Staying Informed and Empowered

Staying informed and empowered is essential for long-term menstrual health and well-being.

Why Staying Informed Matters:

Knowledge is Power: Staying updated with the latest research and information helps you make informed decisions about your health.

Adaptability: Being informed allows you to adapt to changes and new developments in menstrual health.

Empowerment: Knowledge empowers you to take control of your health and advocate for your needs.

Steps to Stay Informed and Empowered:

Empowerment comes from understanding your body, advocating for your needs, and making informed health choices. Below are ways to stay informed and empowered:

1. Continual Learning:

Educational Resources: Regularly read books, articles, and journals on menstrual health.

Workshops and Webinars: Attend workshops and webinars on menstrual health topics.

2. Join Communities:

Support Groups: Stay active in support groups and online communities to share experiences and learn from others.

Professional Networks: Join professional networks related to women's health for more resources and connections.

3. Advocate for Yourself:

Speak Up: Communicate openly with your healthcare provider about your needs and concerns.

Policy Advocacy: Advocate for policies that support menstrual health and access to menstrual products.

4. Stay Positive:

Self-Care: Prioritize self-care and mental well-being as part of your health journey.

Positive Attitude: Maintain a positive attitude towards your menstrual health and body.

> 📢 *Call to Action:* Commit to staying informed and empowered. Continuously seek knowledge, engage with communities, advocate for your health, and maintain a positive outlook.

Key Facts to Remember

✓ *Personal Health Plan:* Creating a personalized menstrual health plan helps you take control of your health and manage your cycle effectively.

✓ *Goal Setting:* Setting specific, measurable, achievable, relevant, and time-bound goals provides direction and motivation.

✓ *Reflection:* Regular reflection helps you understand your progress, learn from your experiences, and make necessary adjustments.

✓ *Continual Learning:* Staying informed about menstrual health and engaging with communities empowers you to make informed decisions and advocate for your needs.

Conclusion

As we come to the conclusion of "Menstrual Health and Management," it's time to reflect on the journey we've undertaken together. This book has been crafted to serve as a comprehensive guide, equipping you with the knowledge, tools, and confidence necessary to navigate your menstrual health journey with clarity and assurance. Let's revisit the major points we've covered to reinforce your understanding and inspire continued empowerment.

Understanding Your Menstrual Cycle

We began by demystifying the menstrual cycle itself, exploring what it is and how it works. You learned about the four phases of the cycle—menstrual, follicular, ovulation, and luteal—and how each phase affects your body and mind. We emphasized the importance of tracking your cycle using apps and techniques to gain insights into your unique patterns and prepare for each phase.

Menstrual Health Essentials

Next, we delved into the anatomy of the female reproductive system, breaking down complex medical terminology into understandable concepts. We discussed the roles of key hormones like estrogen and progesterone and their impact on your cycle. We also covered common menstrual disorders, such as PCOS and endometriosis, providing you with the knowledge to recognize symptoms and seek appropriate medical care when necessary.

Managing Menstrual Symptoms

Managing symptoms is a crucial aspect of menstrual health. We provided practical advice on dealing with cramps through home remedies, medications, and lifestyle changes. For those experiencing heavy periods, we discussed various management strategies and treatments. We also addressed premenstrual syndrome (PMS) and premenstrual dysphoric disorder (PMDD), offering coping mechanisms and holistic approaches to improve your quality of life during these challenging times.

Menstrual Hygiene and Products

Menstrual hygiene is foundational to overall health. We explored the wide range of menstrual products available, from traditional pads and tampons to menstrual cups and reusable options. Best practices for menstrual hygiene were highlighted to prevent infections and ensure comfort. We also looked at eco-friendly products and recent innovations in menstrual care, empowering you to make informed choices that align with your values and lifestyle.

Nutrition and Lifestyle

Your diet and lifestyle play a significant role in your menstrual health. We discussed the importance of a balanced diet, emphasizing foods rich in vitamins and minerals that support your cycle. The positive effects of regular exercise on menstrual health were covered, along with stress management techniques to maintain a healthier cycle. We also examined the benefits of supplements and vitamins in supporting your menstrual health.

Emotional Well-Being

Menstruation is not just a physical experience; it affects your emotional well-being too. We explored the impact of mood swings and emotional changes, offering strategies to manage them through mindfulness and mental health practices. Building a support system and the benefits of journaling and self-reflection were also discussed, highlighting the importance of emotional care during your cycle.

Special Considerations

Different life stages bring unique menstrual health challenges. We addressed the specific needs of adolescents, providing guidance for navigating the onset of menstruation. Menstrual changes during pregnancy and postpartum were discussed, along with what to expect during perimenopause and menopause. For those with chronic conditions, we provided strategies to manage menstrual health effectively.

Breaking the Stigma

Breaking the stigma around menstruation is vital for societal progress. We examined various cultural perspectives on menstruation and advocated for increased awareness and acceptance. Practical advice was given on how to talk to teens about menstrual health and how to create inclusive environments in schools and workplaces, ensuring that menstruation is treated with the respect and normalcy it deserves.

Resources and Support

Finding the right resources and support systems is essential for ongoing menstrual health management. We guided you on how to find the right healthcare provider and the importance of regular medical check-ups. Support groups and online communities were recommended for sharing experiences and gaining support. We also provided a list of recommended reading and educational materials, along with useful apps and tools for tracking and managing your menstrual health.

Your Menstrual Health Journey

Finally, we focused on your personal menstrual health journey. We encouraged you to create a personalized health plan, set specific and achievable goals, and regularly reflect on your progress. Staying informed and empowered is key, and we urged you to continue learning and advocating for your health.

Key Facts to Remember

✓ *Track Your Cycle:* Regular tracking helps you understand and manage your menstrual health better.
✓ *Seek Professional Help*: Regular consultations with healthcare providers ensure you address any issues early.
✓ Manage Symptoms Proactively: Use home remedies, medications, and holistic approaches to manage symptoms effectively.
✓ *Maintain Hygiene:* Choose the right menstrual products and practice good hygiene to prevent infections.
✓ *Adopt a Healthy Lifestyle:* A balanced diet, regular exercise, and stress management contribute to a healthier menstrual cycle.
✓ *Emotional Well-Being Matters:* Address emotional changes with mindfulness, journaling, and a strong support system.
✓ *Understand Life Stage Changes*: Recognize the unique menstrual health needs at different life stages and adapt accordingly.
✓ *Break the Stigma:* Advocate for menstrual health awareness and create inclusive environments.

✓ *Leverage Resources:* Utilize healthcare providers, support groups, and educational materials to stay informed and supported.

Moving Forward

As you move forward, remember that your menstrual health journey is unique. This book is a foundation—a starting point for you to build upon. Continue to educate yourself, seek support, and advocate for your well-being. Embrace your menstrual health with confidence and knowledge, and know that you have the power to manage it effectively.

Thank you for joining me on this journey. Here's to a future of informed, empowered, and confident menstrual health management.

With gratitude and empowerment,

Andrew Henri